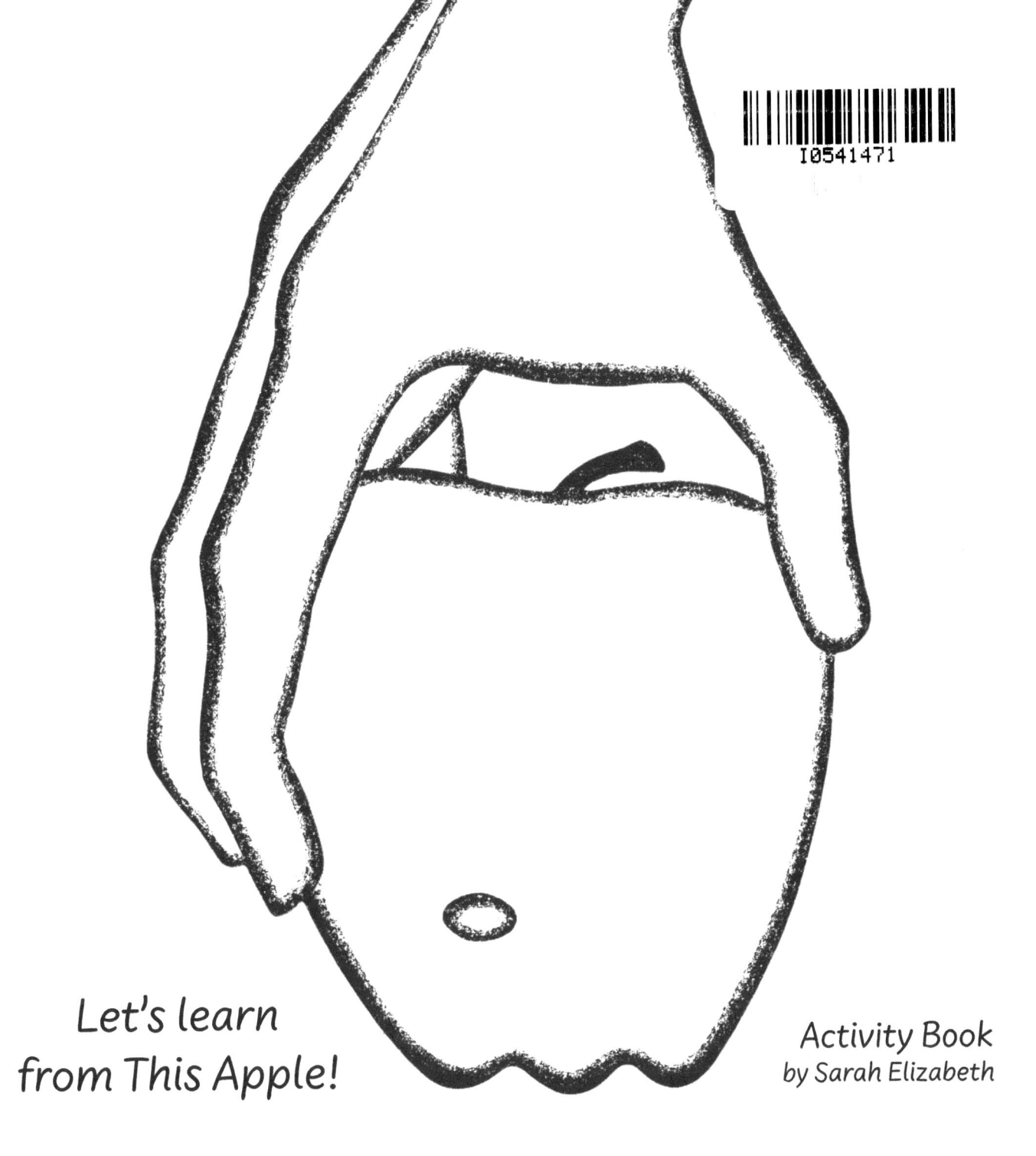

Let's learn
from This Apple!

Activity Book
by Sarah Elizabeth

ISBN: 979-8-9854728-5-1

Published by Sarah Elizabeth
sarah.elizabeth@twinklingsofhope.com

Dear Parents and Guardians,

This activity book is fairly short and purposefully simple, yet hopefully impactful. It's just a starting point, but I wanted to really bring home the message of hope in *This Apple*. This is here for you whenever your child is ready to learn a little more about these topics, provided, of course, that you believe that all of the content is both true and relayed in a helpful way!

Take care!

Sincerely,

Sarah Elizabeth

Can you get this helping hand to the apple?

Draw a line in the path that goes all the way to it!

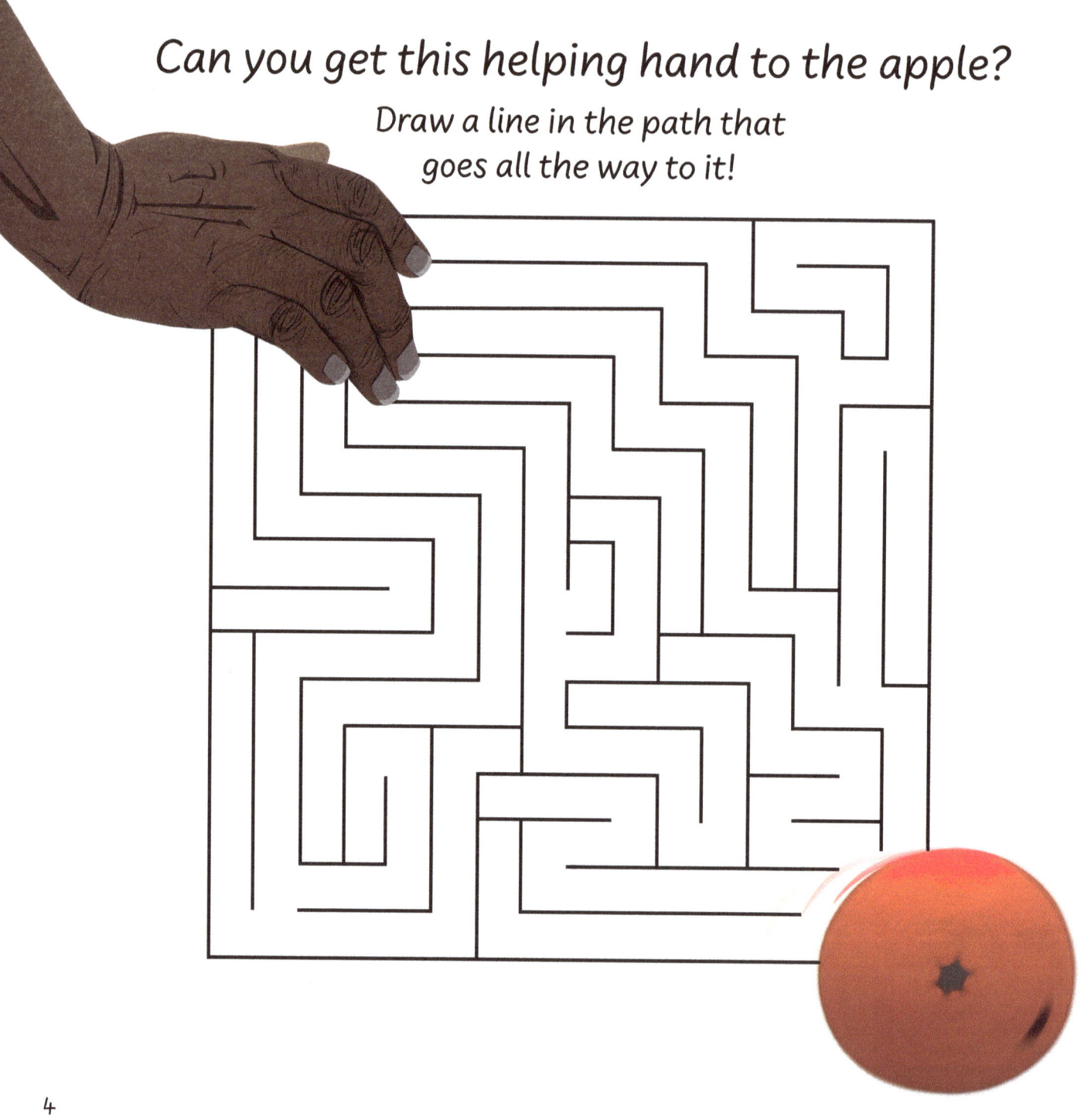

Here's another helping hand from the story!
This is the food bank volunteer's hand.

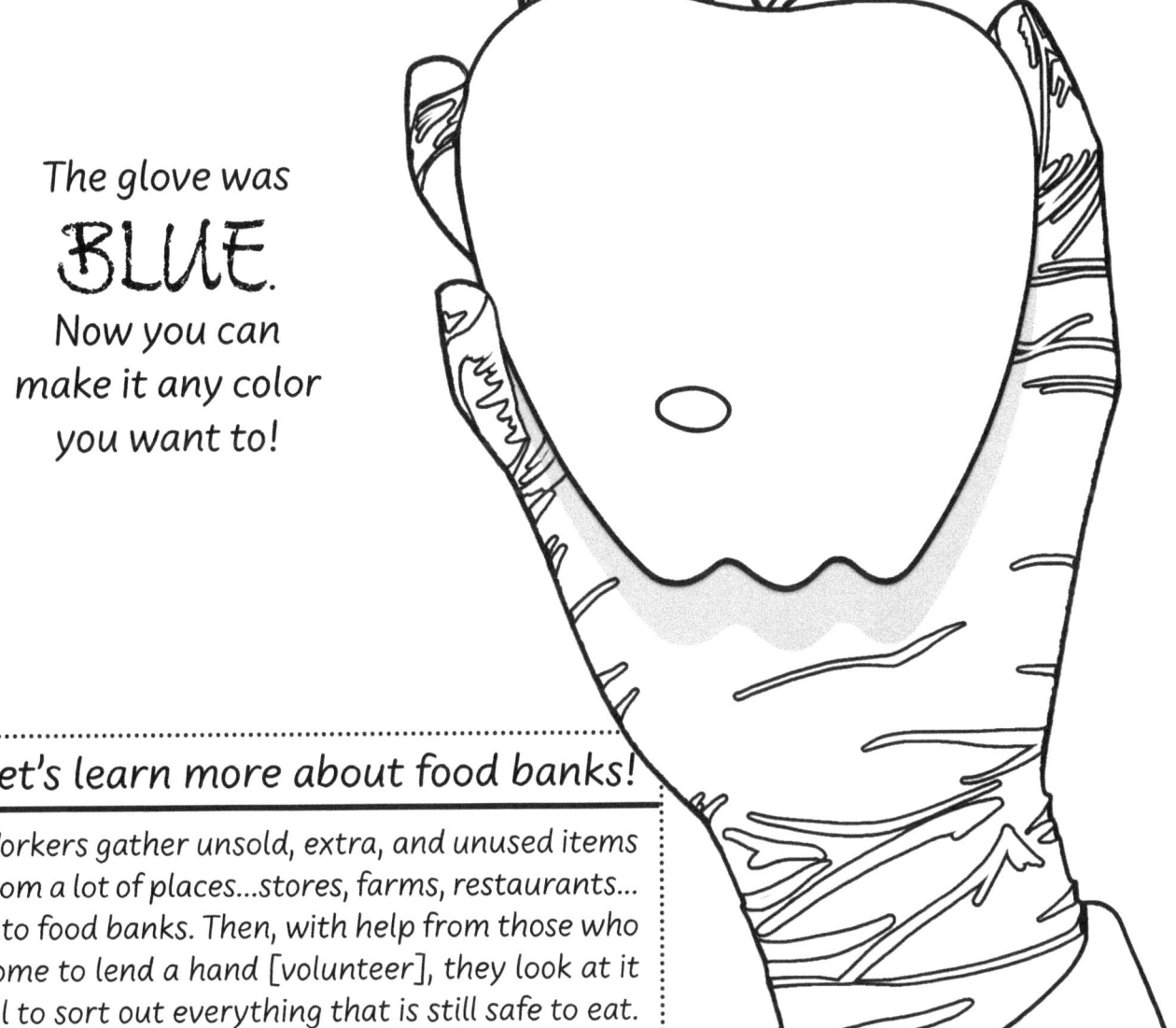

The glove was

BLUE.

Now you can make it any color you want to!

Let's learn more about food banks!

Workers gather unsold, extra, and unused items from a lot of places...stores, farms, restaurants... into food banks. Then, with help from those who come to lend a hand [volunteer], they look at it all to sort out everything that is still safe to eat.

What's different?

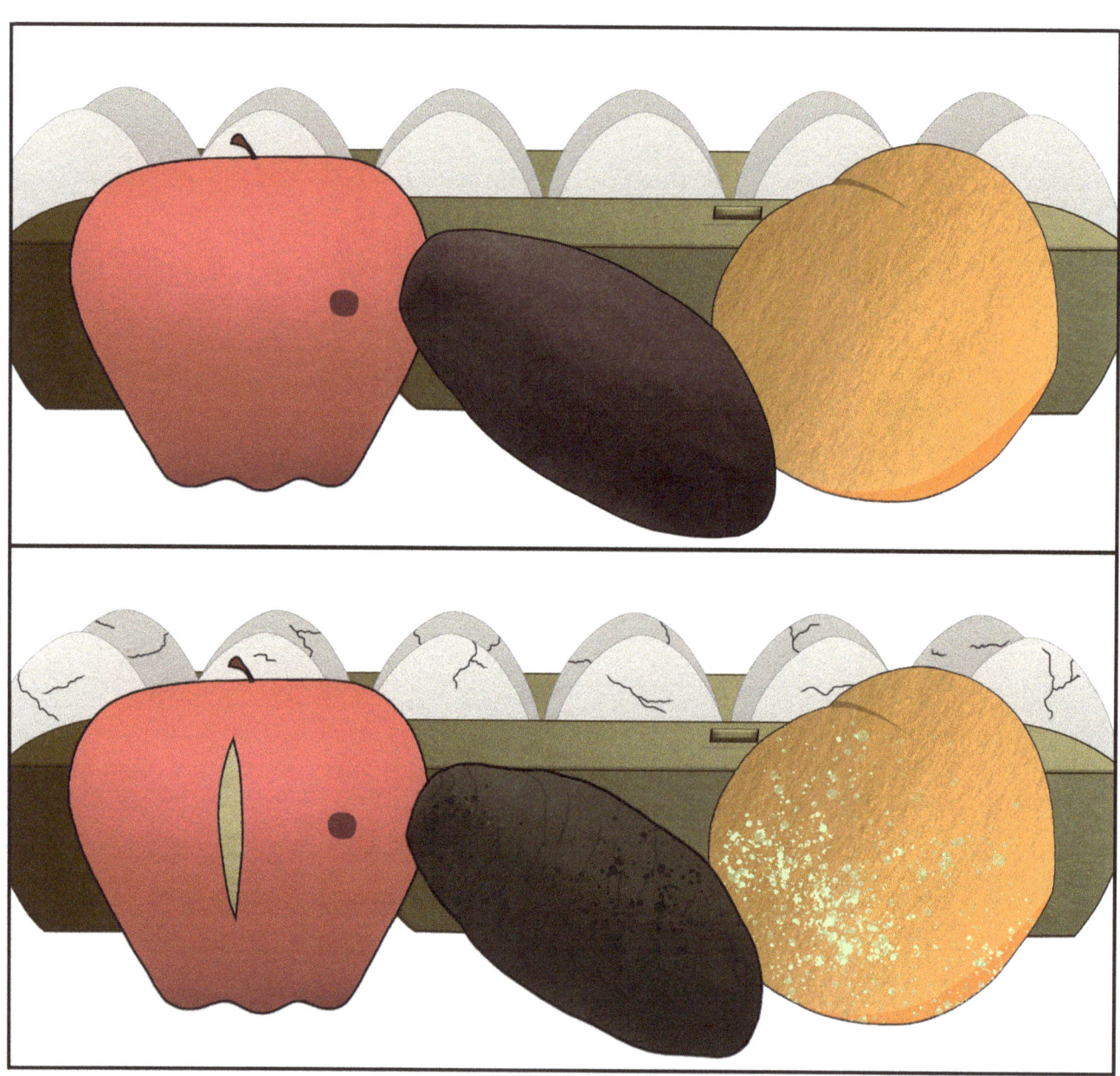

Food does not have to be perfect to be safe to eat, but it should never be...what? Put the broken words back together to find out!

spoiled____   cra_____   spl_____   to_____   mol_____

unse_____   sme_____   sli_____   sti_____   cru_____

dy   lly

~~led~~

my   rn

it   cky

aled

shed   cked

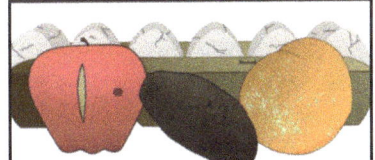

The food in this box is not safe to eat. It would get thrown out.

After being sorted, the safe-to-eat items are sent to food pantries, community kitchens, and other places that also serve people who need help getting enough food and liquids, like milk, for each day.

Draw the missing food in each row's pattern.

It may get harder to fill in as more and more food is missing.
Get help if you need it!

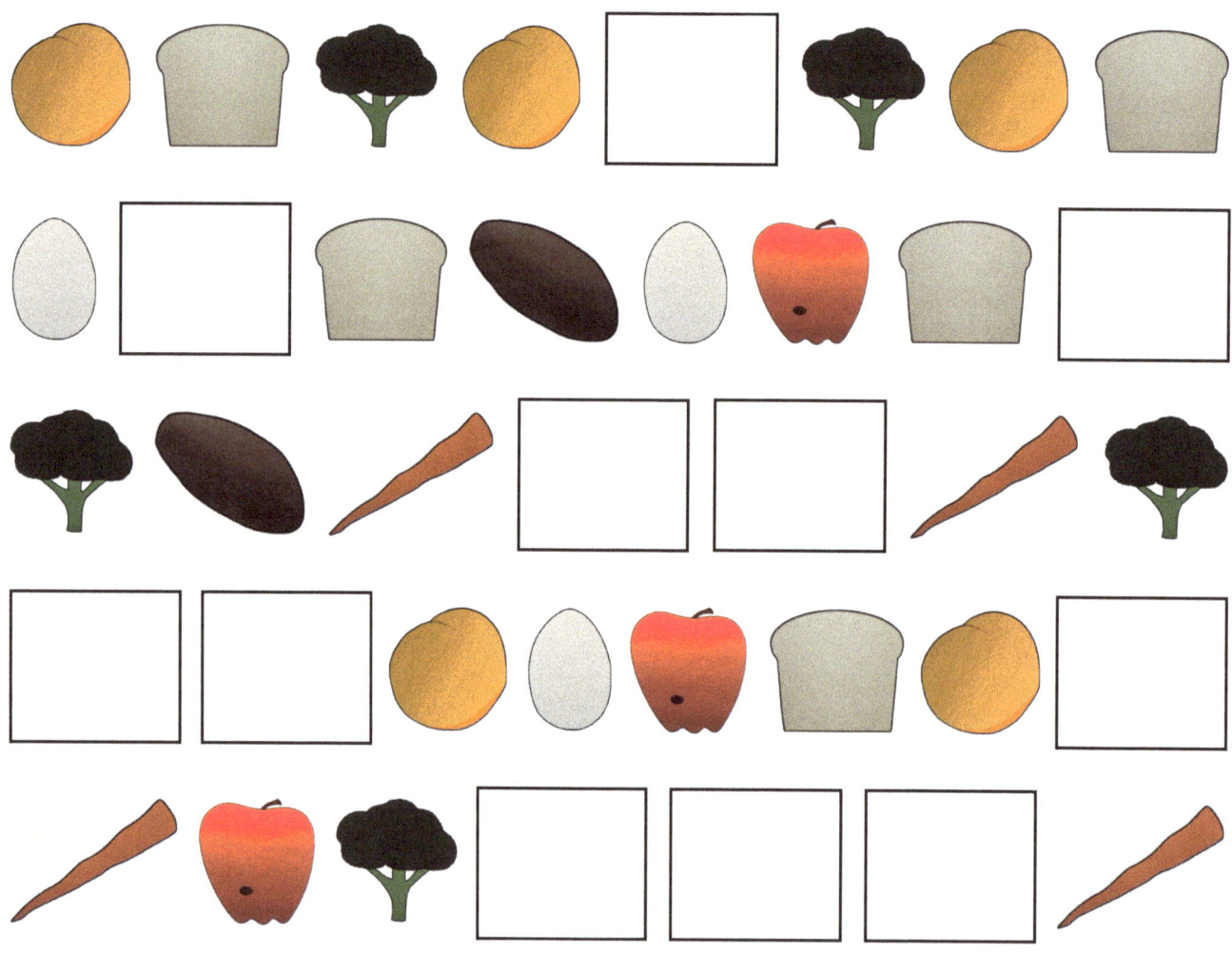

Food helps us grow, think, move, and heal! It's a basic need for life.
If we do not have enough to eat, hunger hurts us more each day.

Many hard things in life can make us need help getting food to eat every day so that we do not stay hungry. These things happen even to people who work hard like this story's mom.

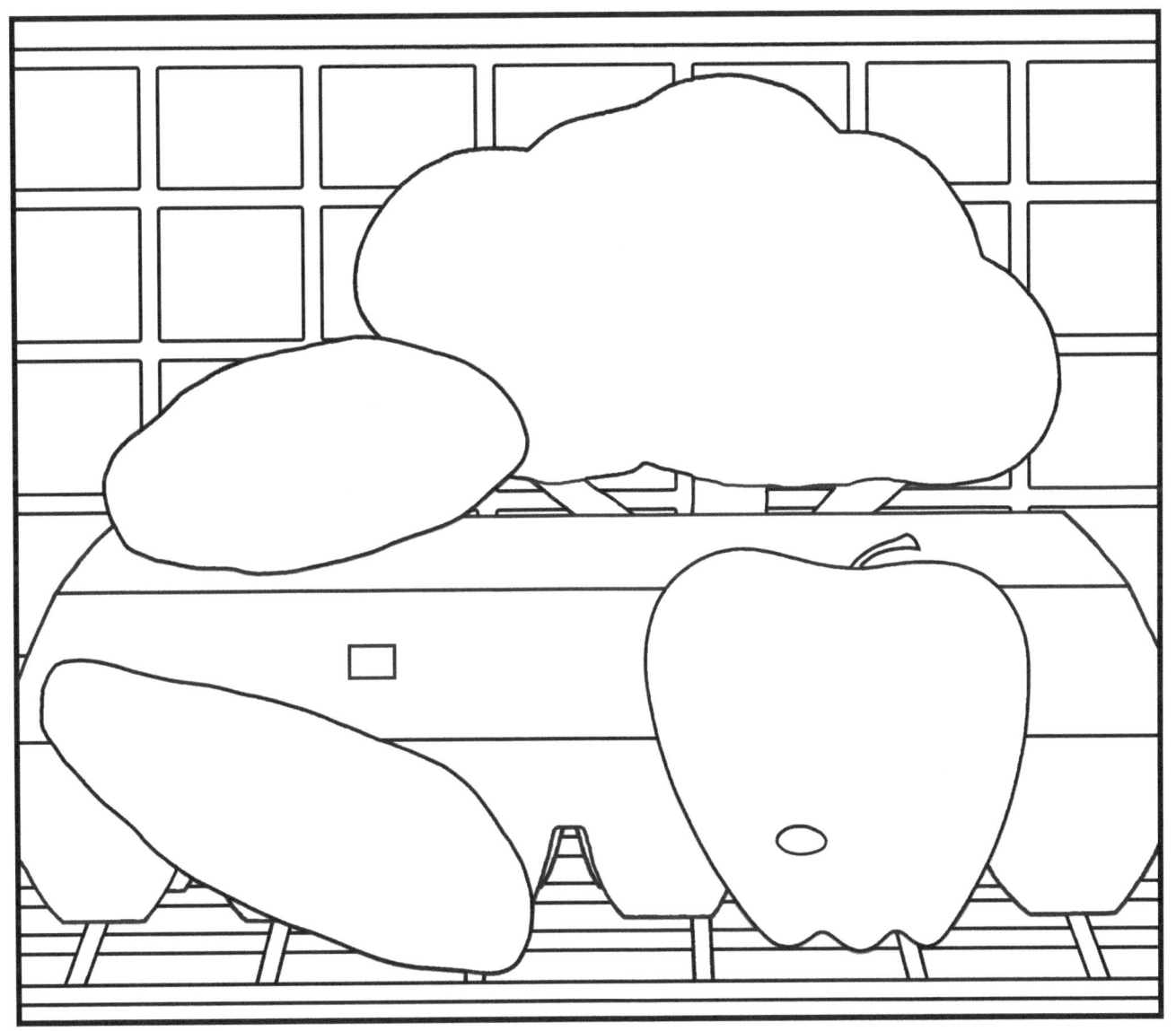

Can you find smaller ones of these in the picture?

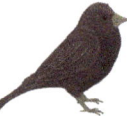 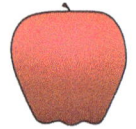 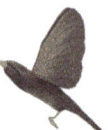

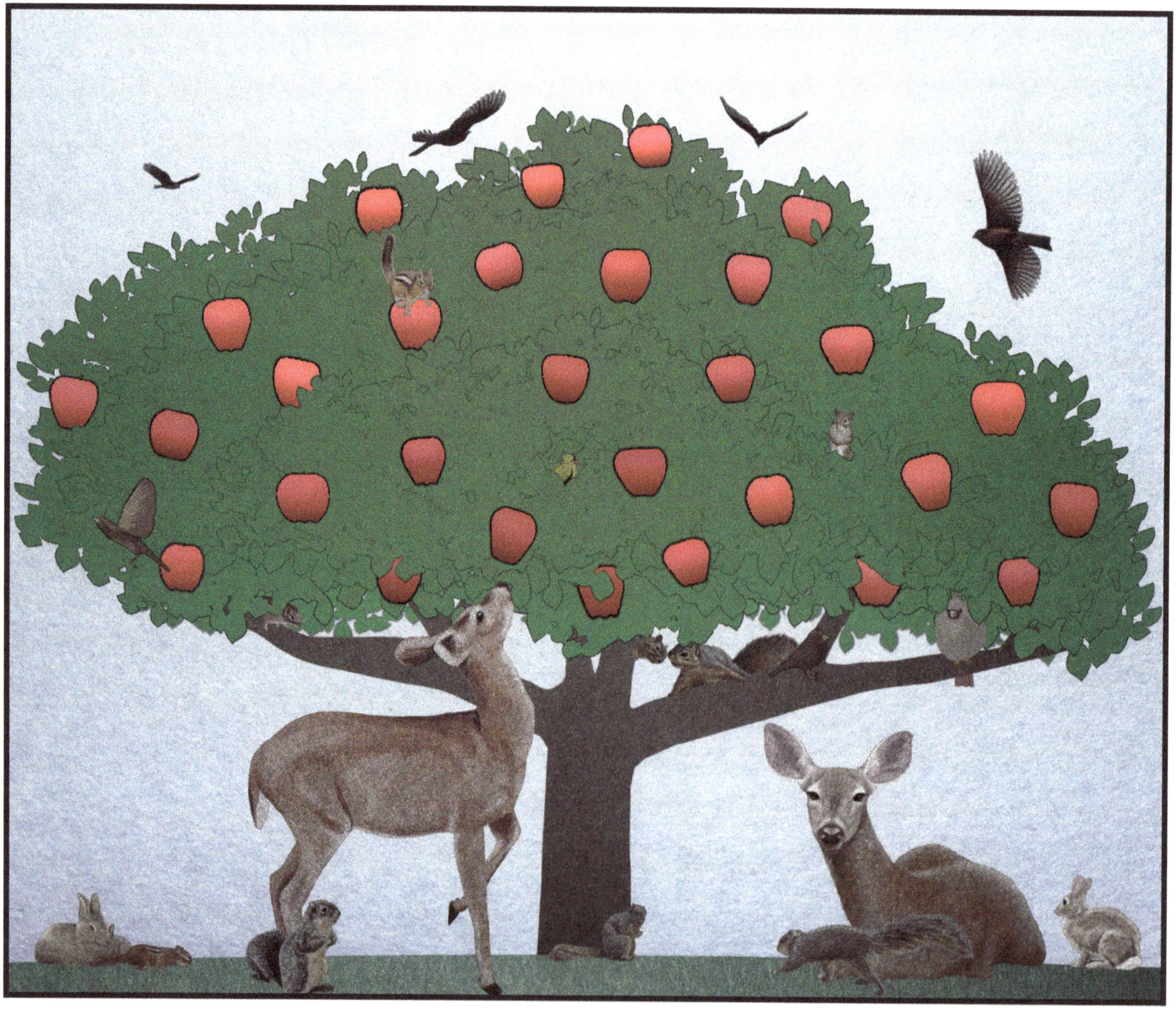

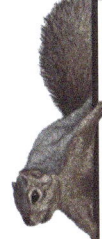

Orchards grow apples for people, so they keep animals away from the fruit. Since this tree is for the animals, there are a lot for you to spot! How many chipmunks, squirrels, bunnies, deer, and other birds do you count?

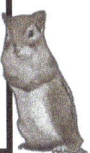

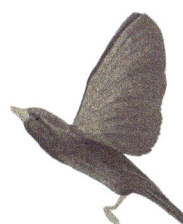

Why are the main things to find that apple and the sparrows?

This tree has so many apples! Finding that one apple's a bit hard. With so many people on the planet, and with so much going on, it is very easy to think that God has the same trouble finding us. But the awesome truth is that God knows exactly where we are! And not just that, God knows all about us and all about our lives. Every detail! Hard times make fear and worry grow, but we can have peace instead, knowing that God loves and takes care of us. Jesus points out God's care even for little sparrows as a reminder that we need not be afraid for we are far more precious to Him!

Can you find this story's apple on the tree?
Here's a hint: it does not have its bruise yet.

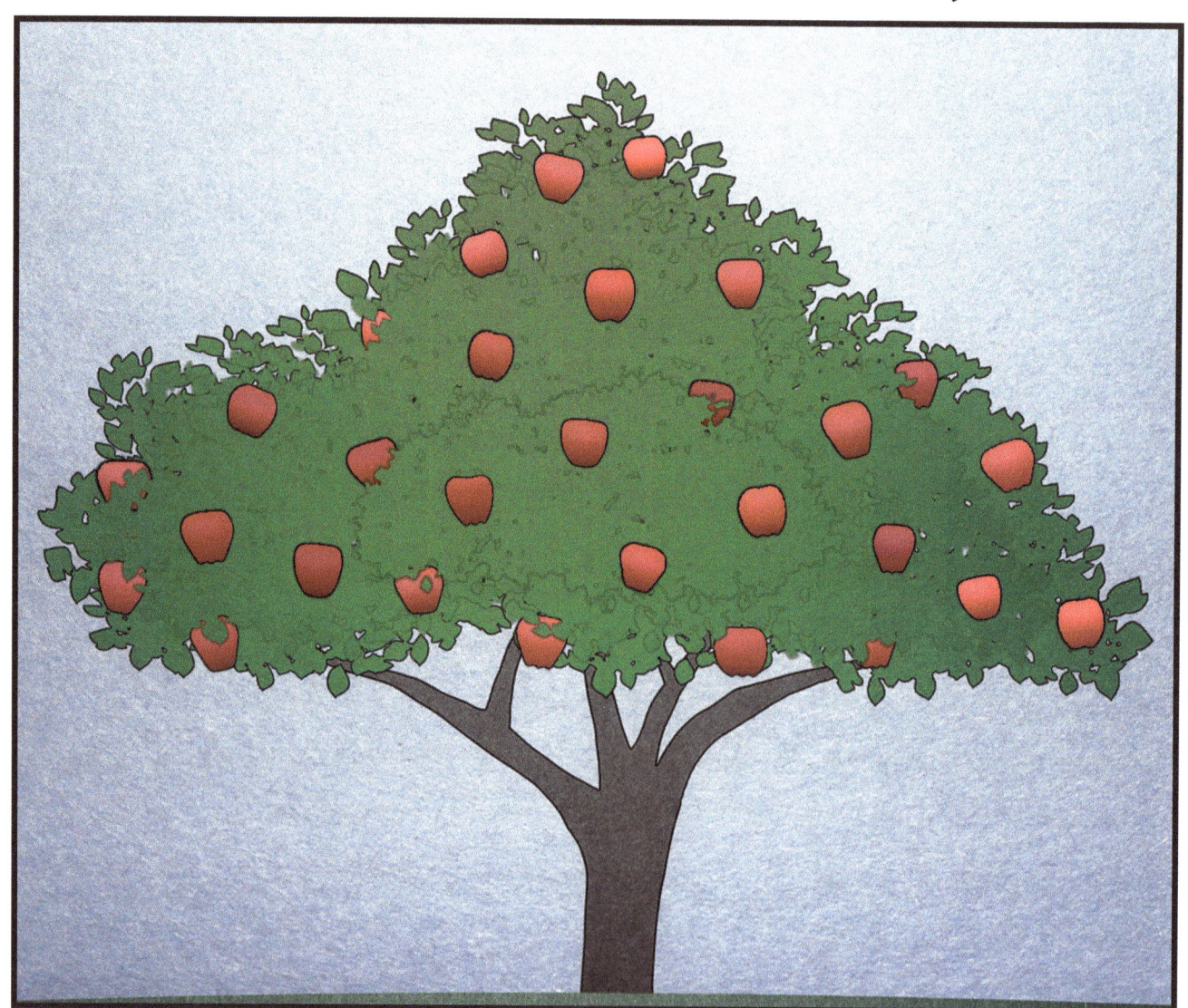

God is at work caring for us long before we have any needs.
Even apple bruises are part of God's good plan to provide...

Can you put these pictures in the right order?
Point to them or mark 1, 2, 3, or 4 in the boxes!

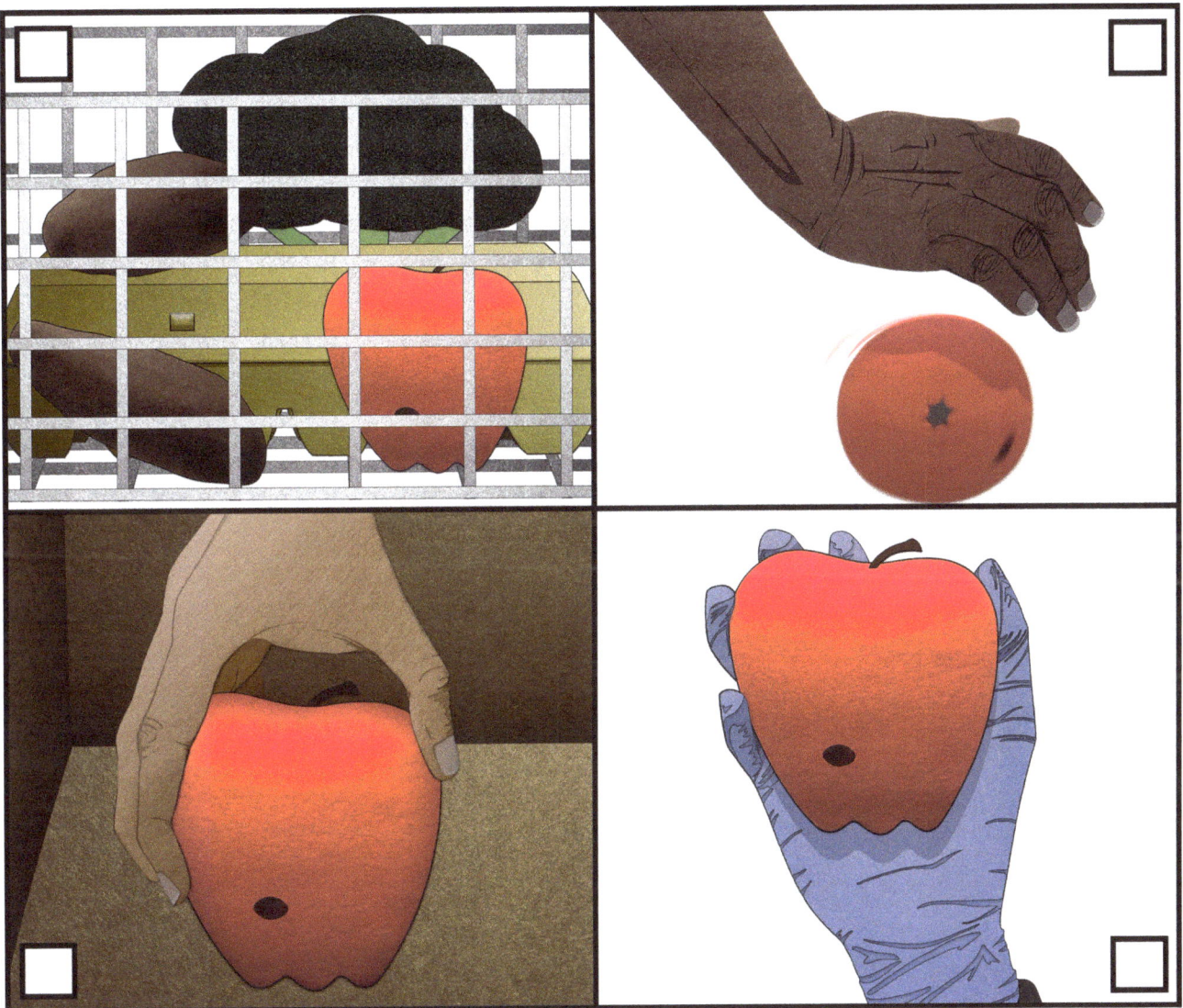

...for God knows how to get what we need to us. God has the love and power to work all things out for His people's good.

God does not promise His people easy lives, but God works all things for the good of whoever will come to believe and trust His Son Jesus.

How and why do we trust God?

We learn who God is and how much He LOVES us through His SON, His Spirit, and the BIBLE, which He has given us to be able to KNOW Him and TRUST our lives to Him, even in really hard times. We learn:

God is GOOD and forgiving.

God has good PLANS for His people.

God wants to and does take CARE of His own.

God abounds in grace, giving us everything we NEED.

God can HELP us with anything. Nothing is too hard for Him.

God has made many PROMISES and He always keeps His word.

TRUST	SON	KNOW	HELP
GOOD	PROMISES	LOVES	
PLANS	BIBLE	NEED	CARE

The words in the box on page 14 can be found in this box.
Circle the ones you find!

P	L	A	N	S	G	V	M	G
R	W	T	R	U	S	T	B	O
O	M	D	K	N	O	W	C	O
M	T	S	B	J	N	E	E	D
I	C	B	I	B	L	E	N	R
S	Y	G	C	R	O	S	S	H
E	K	F	A	M	V	H	K	E
S	U	A	R	W	E	Y	H	L
L	I	F	E	T	S	N	W	P

Two more words that you might find are CROSS and LIFE.

God meant for life to be good, to be full of love and peace and joy, with no one hungry or hurting. It is not that way partly because each of us apart from God does wrong [sins]. Death is the price for sin. But God loves us so His Son Jesus came to conquer sin and pay the price for us by His death on the cross. Jesus did it perfectly. To anyone who turns to Jesus and believes in Him, God gives forgiveness, new life, growth in goodness and more!

We can trust God to one day keep His promise to give eternal life with pure goodness because, unlike with food, which only helps us keep living by coming to its end, Jesus Christ was brought back to life! And from His throne, God ensures our good!

As we wait for God to keep His promise to end all pain and troubles, He is with us and gives us His grace and love to rest in and to share!

Circle the missing piece that fills each picture of active love.

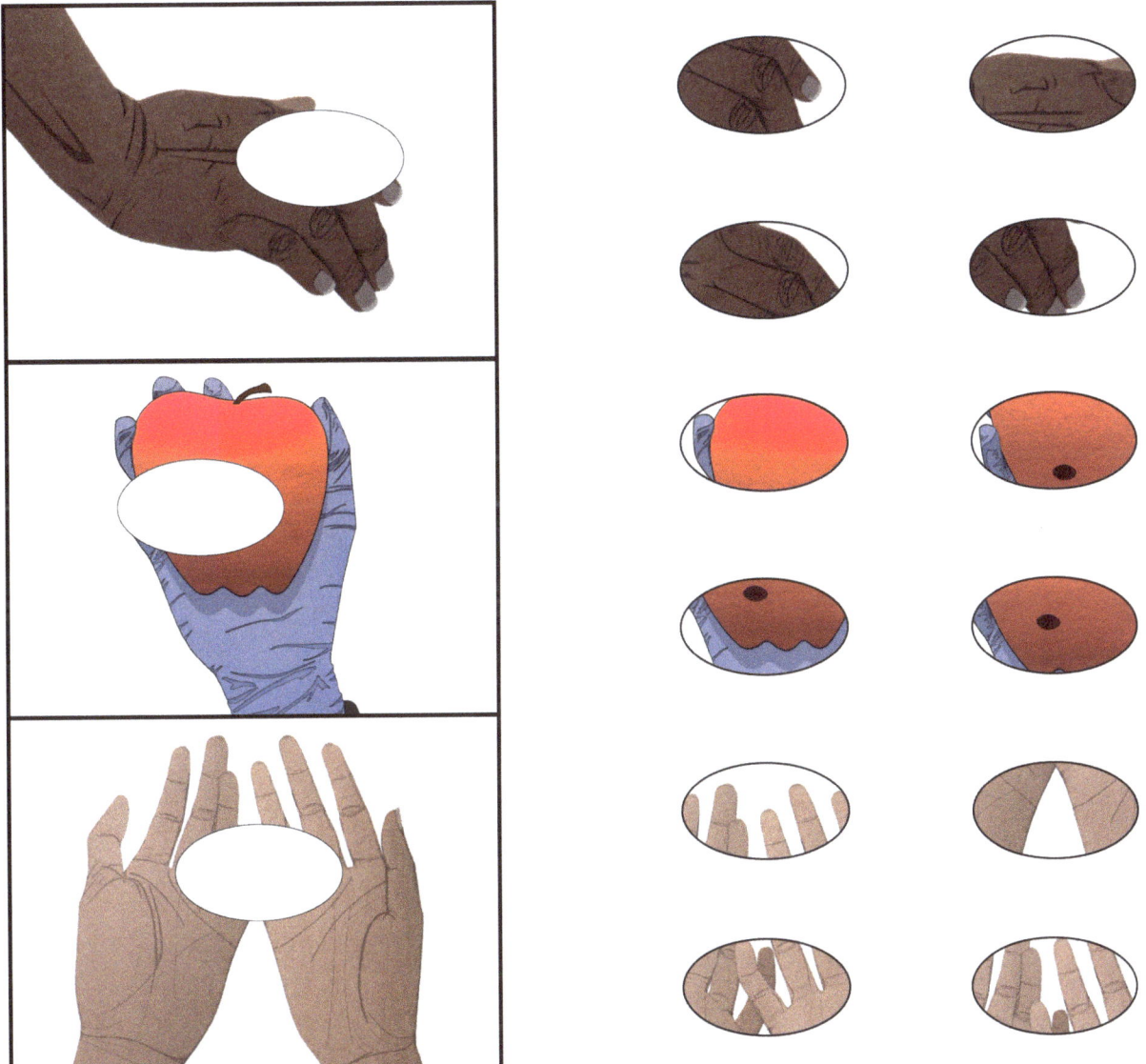

Thank You, God,
for your loving plan for me,
from these hands
all the way back to the tree.